Journey to Holistic Wellness & Weight Loss

This book is intended to share my amazing journey back to holistic wellness, my targeted goal weight, and to inspire others, like you, to view their own journey with a fresh new approach. The most important thing I learned during my challenges and struggles to lose weight, and live a healthier life, was training my mind to accept myself unconditionally, while trusting the process. The most vital components in any successful plan are

Journey to Holistic Wellness & Weight Loss

mental and physical wellness. For many years, I was extremely hard on myself for not fitting in with societies standard of what beauty looked like. It didn't help that I had come up in a family that conformed to the belief that beauty begets wealth, and to achieve success in life I was conditioned to associate with the 'so-called' attractive people. I felt this pressure the most from the male figure in my home, my dad. He was not one to hold

Journey to Holistic Wellness & Weight Loss

his tongue when it came to body shaming my sisters and I, for our physical shortcomings. He subscribed to the stereotype that the most eye pleasing people were the first to be recognized for the highest paying jobs and attracted the wealthiest mates. I believed that I would need physical beauty, to not only survive and be presumed valuable, but to thrive successfully in the world. I never felt good enough, I never felt worthy enough,

Journey to Holistic Wellness & Weight Loss

and thus, I never felt secure in my own body.

I noticeably blossomed into a full-figured girl at a very young age. My earliest years were formed in hiding my curves shamefully, and this was how the road to facing some real battles with my self-esteem began. I had acquired an ideology that was largely built on materialistic, and intangible things, who

Journey to Holistic Wellness & Weight Loss

doesn't want to be happy and fit in well with others? It is a human desire to be a part of a loving, and supportive community of family and friends. I believed that for a woman to live well, to a ripe old age, she had to be two things, attractive and strategically submissive. Catching the eye of some prince on a white horse was a dream told through hearing fairytales stories written by dreamers. Living a happy, and abundant

Journey to Holistic Wellness & Weight Loss

life wouldn't necessarily require me to have the highest form of education, or years of valuable work experience, or even be a positive role model for society. All I had to do was focus on my outside appearances, and my inside approach, what an artificial mindset! I will admit, although, that my parents did endorse a college education as an added plus, as well as a few other achievements. They were presented as more of a buffer than a means

Journey to Holistic Wellness & Weight Loss

to survive or thrive. It was subliminally expressed that, as a woman, especially a black woman living in a patriarchal world, I should be realistic about how high I set my long-term goals. Thus, I set my goals on obtaining a husband, who was a protector, and preferably a gainfully employed one. To achieve this goal, it would be important to keep my body in good shape, grow my hair long (keeping it pressed straight, not naturally kinky), and

Journey to Holistic Wellness & Weight Loss

to remember not to speak when a man was speaking; that was a woman's time to learn. Pretty old-fashioned thinking, and quite nauseating when I look back on it. You'd be surprised how many young girls still face this type of male influence in their homes today. They too are brainwashed by fathers praying for the highest bidder to come and ask for their daughter's hand in marriage. Their goal is to be free from the burden of feeding and

Journey to Holistic Wellness & Weight Loss

clothing her. So young girls are molded to be good, disciplined wives, and prepared to live in a man's world, with a closed mouth and open legs. You can find these patriarchal practices all over the world today, still, in just about every culture, every religion, every work sector, and in every community. Systematic and subliminal messages are used to control the 'divine feminine' from rising and claiming her rightful place in the world.

Journey to Holistic Wellness & Weight Loss

The conditioning usually begins early in life and may last for years.

I remember dreaming of one day being admired, desired, and considered worthy of being swept off my feet. I wanted to be part of the highly valued groups like the women I saw on television, and in the magazines. I needed to fit in somewhere. Marriage was a must, according to my parents, and I strived to

Journey to Holistic Wellness & Weight Loss

connecting with a hard-working man who could take charge in running a well-organized home. He, of course, would be a church going man who claimed to fear God and love his bible. I know how this all may sound, so far, stick with me the rabbit hole goes deeper. I truly was a slave to the judgments of others, and the negative conditioning of an ancient mindset.

Journey to Holistic Wellness & Weight Loss

It seemingly was not a bad trade, beauty for long term security, and how hard could it be to achieve? Then one day, out of nowhere, some very noticeable changes took place, uncontrollably. I got a stroke of good luck when I was chosen to attend High school far from my home, not in my zoned area. I would be allowed to travel a longer distance from home to school every day. Now into my teens I could venture out solo more, and more. In

Journey to Holistic Wellness & Weight Loss

my daily travels to and from school (my sisters and I chose to attend different schools, at this point) I found exposure to other people, of different cultures. I was open to learning and engaging in real life conversations with educators (mostly women, to my surprise), young people my age, and an array of different perspectives on life. I had been sheltered for so long, my brain, and my soul craved excitement. I could now hear my own inner voice loudly and it was screaming for adventure.

I did notice one startling thing. The reactions on the faces of others, just by listening to all the brainwashing I had undergone at home, were a bit embarrassing, and I quickly knew I was carrying some demons. The world began to look very different; I questioned everything I knew. It was like I was handed a big bowl of new and exciting colorful options. The universe was gifting

Journey to Holistic Wellness & Weight Loss

me with a free pass to choose a new direction, with a fresh new set of eyes. I then decided it was time to work on my self-confidence, be open to making some big changes, and invite some new positive connections into my small bubble.

There were so many things I could do now attending school, so I joined the dance team, the cheerleading team, and played volleyball at school; anything that

Journey to Holistic Wellness & Weight Loss

could keep me in good shape and allow me to feel good in my growing body. This was also a good way to make friends and stay inclusive. I was intending to kill a few birds with one stone by adding in some cardio exercise that would ensure I would hold my place in line; obviously still stuck in that body shaming frequency, I wore myself out to say the least! I also attended study groups to keep my grades up, joined afterschool clubs, and was

Journey to Holistic Wellness & Weight Loss

determined to build my own happier place,

away from home. I became a social

butterfly and noticed that the people I

hung around didn't seem to care about my

physical appearance, as much as they

cared about my personality. This

prompted me to take a closer look at the

religious and moral values that my parents

preached. For years, my siblings and I had

been subjected to long hours and multiple

days attending church services, functions,

Journey to Holistic Wellness & Weight Loss

and related events. "Jesus" was proudly named the head of our home by my dad, who was an honored deacon, and a mason; had to mention that! My mother was a silent homemaker who followed the male standard promoted in our home. Father ran a tight ship and mom made sure it was always clean, presentable to others, and a picture of the perfect family; it wasn't. Soon enough my sisters and I grew out of needing her motherly supervision, and

Journey to Holistic Wellness & Weight Loss

then mother was influenced (by our dad) to get a full-time job and help pay the bills. I was completely baffled and lost! Father had me believing that a woman's work was in the home, and that her man's job was to go out and provide for her and his children. Yet as soon as his need for her changed he was happy to throw her to the wolves and have her survive in a world she was not prepared for, to help him accomplish his financial responsibilities.

Journey to Holistic Wellness & Weight Loss

Once again, I took a long-term look at marriage, at the behavior of men, and their genuine need of having a woman in the home, in a different light.

Moving on, and now attending my senior year of high school, I decided it was time to try finding a part-time job. I wanted to get a taste of the working world and test my new independent nature. I grew tired of asking my parents for a

Journey to Holistic Wellness & Weight Loss

hand-out that came with a lecture about gratitude and priorities. I had learned a lot about who I was and what I wanted, from being around others, throughout my scholastic experience. "One day I would work in a corporation, as a front office representative like a secretary, or an administrative assistant", that was where I could see myself the happiest. Back then women appeared to be placed in positions where they could attract incoming traffic

Journey to Holistic Wellness & Weight Loss

for business. I now liked meeting and greeting new people, and I fancied being in the spotlight; again, killing two birds with one stone. I could be recognized while making my own wage. My confidence had grown although I still struggled silently with the idea of being beautiful, and worthy in the eyes of the beholder. My parents had created a self-sabotaging, co-dependent, and toxic mindset in me by feeding me all the

Journey to Holistic Wellness & Weight Loss

glamour and rewards of people pleasing, and school didn't completely erase all those years of molding. I had been engrossed in this system of belief for so long it would take a lot of inner work to change it. Determined to push through the negative inner voices and get a victory for myself, married or single, rich, or poor, accepted or rejected kept me on the move. I found that there was no one who could love me better than I could, thus I started

Journey to Holistic Wellness & Weight Loss

to believe more and more in myself.   I
knew, at this point, that something about
me was different than the others in my
home. I was more of a rebel and wasn't
afraid to be alone, a lot.   There was a fire
deep down in my bones that was not
taught to me but seemed divinely guided
by a mysterious source. I was a lonely
wanderer searching for a bigger meaning
to why I existed on this planet, and
moreover in this family that seemed like

Journey to Holistic Wellness & Weight Loss

an alien nation. I refused to fear the unknown burdens of being independent, as much as I was told too. There was always a light at the end of the tunnel and I knew that if I just kept taking the journey, paying attention to the red flags, and seeking a bigger me, that I would fall upon my path to success and happiness.

I wasn't sure if college would happen right after high school. My parents

Journey to Holistic Wellness & Weight Loss

promoted a college education but did not prepare, financially, for any of us to attend. They did not save any money to help my sisters or I, nor had any plans as to how we could achieve obtaining a degree. It appeared that all those days and nights on our knees, praying for financial miracles and breakthroughs, were for show. The adults didn't practice what they preached. What was really the point of spending all that time worshipping, I

Journey to Holistic Wellness & Weight Loss

thought? I saw my father, for years, give more to a building full of lost souls (the church) than he received. Where were all the blessings the parishioners claimed were a guaranteed reward for obedience to the faith! I watched the pastors' sons successfully complete college, debt free. I watched his family go on yearly vacations, drive fancy cars, and live in a beautiful home, all financed by funds collected from the church, donated by a struggling

Journey to Holistic Wellness & Weight Loss

congregation, desperate for life-changing miracles to show up and change their lives too.   Church became just another system of slavery and bondage; ciphering energy, time, money, and hope from unsuspecting, low income, poverty stricken, and I hate to say it, but poorly educated minorities.

It was time to make my own rules, my own decisions, and start moving away from religious based and societal

Journey to Holistic Wellness & Weight Loss

stereotypes. My first decision was to take a year or two off from attending college after high school, maybe work a bit, save up some money, and see more of the world. My parents had never traveled outside of the US, when I was growing up, and I wanted to experience life everywhere. Depending on human contact as confirmation that I was relatable, likeable, and accepted was still a battle internally. Still, silently, struggling with

Journey to Holistic Wellness & Weight Loss

self-esteem issues I focused more on strengthening my positive connections. Those inner toxic voices were always waiting in the wind to remind me of my limitations so it was important to keep my mind busy on healthier affirmations. It was a lot of pressure, for a young girl, to worry so much about how to navigate her own future but what choice did I have? Life hadn't afforded me a map to "the yellow brick road"; I surely felt like I was

Journey to Holistic Wellness & Weight Loss

Dorothy in the Wizard of Oz seeking a brain though!

All those years of physical activity, in school, had made my full-figured body more curvy and more noticeable, and the men (and women) started to notice me in a more intimate way. Initially I welcomed the attention, and the reassuring compliments about how attractive I was. The voices were very different from the judgements I had come to know at home.

I must mention, for a better mental picture,

that my sisters were not so lucky,

physically, and it caused some noticeable

envy and jealousy when we were growing

up, and I was bullied by them publicly, for

years. When out with friends, in schools

we attended together, at large family

events, and even at church they never

missed an opportunity to make negative

references to my 'big booty', my dark

complexion skin, or the hypnotizing giggle in my walk. I was called names like blacky, fatty, big booty Lucy, Bertha butt, and so on, you get the point. They claimed that the only reason the boys wanted me was for a quickie, or to get a squeeze of my goodies. My first intimate connections were not good ones, as you can tell. All it did was cause me to not trust boys, or any male frankly! I felt like aliens from outer space dropped on the

Journey to Holistic Wellness & Weight Loss

wrong planet, in the wrong century. With no close emotional support and no one to confide in about what I was experiencing inside my mental space, I learned to internalize every painful encounter. I am sure you can understand the importance of having healthy role models in life, especially for a child, male or female. I grew up wondering if something was wrong with me, or if my life was a cruel joke, and if this was how it would always

Journey to Holistic Wellness & Weight Loss

be. No one else in the house looked the way I did, behaved the way I did, spoke the way I did, wanted the things I did, and it began to be a sore spot in my ego. What was I supposed to do about the body I inherited or that God chose me to have? At this point I even questioned why God put me in this body, with this family, in this lifetime, on this planet. "Jesus" was deemed the head of our home but I felt like His "forgotten child". Where was

Journey to Holistic Wellness & Weight Loss

Christ when I needed Him; the man I was told who loved and favored the innocent children, and the pure of heart? I had been emotionally abandoned and rejected by my own family for no apparent reason. How many of you can relate to that? Whether it is or was about weight, culture, ethnicity, religion, gender, status, envy, jealousy, greed, or a lack of human empathy, many of you can relate to a time where you felt judged by others or didn't

Journey to Holistic Wellness & Weight Loss

fit in with your own family. I learned that the exposure of a toxic family was a hinderance to finding a heathy independence and freedom from environmental slavery; my life so far was the textbook version.

Having finished high school and securing a part-time job, here and there I found it easier to ignore my inner battles. It was easier to stay in the streets, working

Journey to Holistic Wellness & Weight Loss

meaningless jobs, then be happy at home or attending college. I made a little money for myself and I could pursue my traveling and bigger goals in life, which were to live freely to do the things that brought me some joy. A plus would be to do it while looking great and feeling appreciated though. Eventually landed a full-time job and started looking for a way to move out of my parents' house. I knew I had no time for self-pity and couldn't waste time

Journey to Holistic Wellness & Weight Loss

on what was going on inside my emotional and mental space. I labeled every struggle as 'growing pains' and hoped for the best. I battled every day with what I saw in the mirror but wouldn't let (her) stop me. I was not a picture of the perfect tall, lean, and slender woman my father raved about on television, and I probably was never going to be. By now, I had stopped dancing and playing sports. Slowly my firmness really began to wiggle and giggle

Journey to Holistic Wellness & Weight Loss

a little more. I remained focused on working, saving money, and obtaining my own place. I had to build an egg full of money to do so because I was used to upper middle-class living and planned on continuing to do so. Working, on my feet mostly, was becoming an issue physically because of the weight I slowly accumulated. I started calling out sick more often, from being sore and tired. Like most Americans I was consuming

Journey to Holistic Wellness & Weight Loss

lots of fast food instead of mother's home cooking, which wasn't very healthy either but I'll get to that in a minute. Soon, I was back to asking my well-off dad for money to hang out with friends. My dad always had more than enough to spend but made you beg for it, or what he called 'earn it'! I figured I had done what I was told to do by finishing high school, securing some means of financial support for myself, and graduating high school. Yet it was never

Journey to Holistic Wellness & Weight Loss

enough to please a father who seemed determined to keep me small, and dependent on him. I knew I had some obvious circumstances that were working against me. To gain the income necessary to live on my own, snag the perfect higher paying job, and a great potential helpmate, I had to change my stinking thinking and do something about my overall declining health. The mounting weight and the lack of physical activity was causing me to

Journey to Holistic Wellness & Weight Loss

slow down and stay indoors more, depression began to set in, and my insecurities increased 10-fold. I was still so young but mentally so engrossed in adult issues. I was barely out of high school and was hyper focused on a future, that looked bleak. Why couldn't I simply focus on dating, living a youthful life of having fun, and experiencing who I could be in the world; you know, being a young person, still living at home, and supported

Journey to Holistic Wellness & Weight Loss

by a loving family. What happened to my fairy tale story of growing from a child into an adult, while enjoying a beautiful life with no expectations and no restrictions, simply living wild and free; at least that was my fairy tale dream. My inner feminine goddess, as I came to recognize her, was desperate for change. She had dreams of being released onto the world, full of passion for life, and a thirst to experience more than I'd been handed

Journey to Holistic Wellness & Weight Loss

so far. All the misguided teachings, church rules, and patriarchal discipline that had been constantly etched in my mind, by a father who believed he was my savior, and a mother who was complacent or just mentally tuned out, had eaten a hole in my soul. I was long overdue for a "conscious shift", that could save my life.

Moving on, now eighteen years old, I lost my virginity to my high school

Journey to Holistic Wellness & Weight Loss

sweetheart.   It was not a fairy tale experience y'all, LOL! *I got pregnant, on my first-time having sex,* the universe must have truly hated me, I thought. OMFG is right, I couldn't get a break. Unfortunately for me, no one had guided me into a healthy transition from adolescence to womanhood, safely. My mother never spoke to any of us about sex, birth control, std's, or anything that made her uncomfortable, or considered ungodly. I

Journey to Holistic Wellness & Weight Loss

assumed my father believed she had since she only birthed girls. It surely wasn't going to be a conversation he had with us. I guess my sisters and I were supposed to learn about sex and caring for our female reproductive systems in school by strangers. You'd think we could turn to the elder woman at church, right? Church also didn't provide the answers I needed instead I was plagued with constant scolding about being obedient and

Journey to Holistic Wellness & Weight Loss

disciplined, and fed one-sided ancient ideologies that were grounded in the shame of being born into sin. Once my dad found out I was no longer a virgin, by the pediatrician who confirmed I was pregnant, at a scheduled physical, I was immediately scheduled for an abortion. No church going man of God, a deacon of the church, could allow a 'bastard' baby to stain his reputation. My mother was more sensitive to my situation but could not find

Journey to Holistic Wellness & Weight Loss

father and to stand up for me, against my father, and let me choose what was right for me and my unborn baby. All she could do was cry silently for me, as I heard her doing one night while she prayed. Soon after, the secret was buried, and I was seemingly restored to a vision of purity. I would then be forced to take birth control pills to avoid another disgraceful situation for my parents. My sisters were elated with the whole belittling situation, of

Journey to Holistic Wellness & Weight Loss

course, and I listened to them gloat and snicker at my shame. Our parents made sure that while we lived in their home, we added to the illusion that it was a holy and sanctified place; it was more like my hell. The deacon didn't shy away from abortion as an option as soon as his reputation as a perfect father was in jeopardy; once again I was lost, but not surprised. Enraged by the lies, deception, and betrayal to walk in the spirit of God gave me great pause!

Journey to Holistic Wellness & Weight Loss

Even with the masks being torn off the biggest benefit of being exposed to a spiritual connection, with The Highest, was that I learned how to channel some inner strength, through meditation and prayer. There's that mysterious divine source I mentioned earlier. I would admit that all these negative life experiences made me question if God was listening at all sometimes though. Did I really need Him as the head of my life, if He wasn't

Journey to Holistic Wellness & Weight Loss

showing up for me? My faith was diminishing and my heart was heavy, the world was dark and cold. I begged God to talk to me and tell me why this was all happening to me? I just sat and waited for an answer.

I soon discovered that birth control pills were highly recommended to young girls as the easiest guard against unwanted pregnancy. They had been introduced to

Journey to Holistic Wellness & Weight Loss

me without any regard for their pros and cons to my still developing body. I was not advised to review the side effects or research past patient reviews related to the pill prescribed to me. Neither my physician, nor my parents considered that I was too young to seek this information out on my own; my mother had never been exposed to this modern medication and could not guide me in any way. Consuming these pills proved to be an

Journey to Holistic Wellness & Weight Loss

instrument of harm to my body, both hormonally and physically, thus emotionally and mentally. Just what I needed! I was already battling the self-hate I felt after getting pregnant out of wedlock, shaming my parents, and aborting a life that I had felt God placed in me for a bigger purpose, possibly to beak some obvious generational curses. Consuming these pills for years led to experiencing many health challenges, both

Journey to Holistic Wellness & Weight Loss

while taking them and when finally trying to come off them.   *This is not to deter any 'woman' from considering this form of birth control. * "I will say that I found that there were safer, long-term options, that should have been presented to me." Using condoms would not only have been safer, health-wise, they would have also been a deterrent to STD exposure; the pill did not achieve this. At a time where my body was going through many challenges

Journey to Holistic Wellness & Weight Loss

internally and externally, I also lacked exposure to energetic, nutritional, and healing food(s). Growing up in a world of processed junk foods, fast foods, and life-on-the-go eating habits was popular and easier to maintain monetarily. Eating a diet of whole foods, organically grown, and ethically sourced was way more expensive and harder to find. Nutritionally, I was diving deeper into disaster every day and lessoning my

Journey to Holistic Wellness & Weight Loss

lifespan along the way. Like many young people living in a big city my time moving about day-to-day resembled a replay of consuming unhealthy food and beverages. Images were being flashed across all media platforms directly targeting young people to enjoy eating fast, easily obtainable, and on-the-go meals. It appeared that the government was keeping generations of enslaved zombies living a pre-destined, fast-paced, constantly busy,

Journey to Holistic Wellness & Weight Loss

materialistic, and immediate gratification seeking lifestyle. A goal to keep people working, paying taxes, chasing a dream of owning their own home, and unfocused on their overall health was subliminally portrayed. A culture of profitable disease carriers was being manifested and mass produced. Enticing visuals of delicious and popular dishes like stuffed pizzas, loaded burgers, greasy chicken spots, sweetened sugary drinks, and deep-fried

Journey to Holistic Wellness & Weight Loss

treats were on billboards, at bus stops, train stations, near schools, playgrounds, medical facilities, and even by the hospitals, and the cemeteries, go figure! You can find them still existing today, there's a huge industry promoting fast food options at lower costs than fresh fruits and vegetables consistently. You can also expect to see a flow of weight loss formulas to combat obesity and the diseases associated with unhealthy eating

Journey to Holistic Wellness & Weight Loss

habits, posted nearby, mind blowing. I questioned why most diseases in the body are labeled as 'hereditary'. Instead, they should be listed as 'acquired' when the diets that lead to them are promoted for the financial gain of an economy. Obesity was a growing market scheme for the industry to increase funds to produce more diseases to treat, growing more income for the internal revenue services

Journey to Holistic Wellness & Weight Loss
(the wealthy in-charge), that's how I saw

it. In contrast,

the magazines and media outlets were

constantly depicting happy looking,

aesthetically beautiful, and unnaturally

thin men and women as role models. The

messages being put out were confusing,

and misleading, and proved that there was

an obvious unspoken agenda. Even

though models represented a very small

Journey to Holistic Wellness & Weight Loss
fraction of people in the world I couldn't

get away from what society deemed

beautiful and coveted it. The desire to

become what my eyes caught in the rear-

view mirror, while giving a lot of attention

to getting money, and keeping the pace

with society was killing my spirit. The

money these people obtained, especially

the women models, had afforded them an

extravagant lifestyle that I wanted.

Journey to Holistic Wellness & Weight Loss
Women like that had the luxury of what

seemed to be a self-reliant lifestyle. How

wonderful it would be to not have to ask

anyone for anything? All I knew was that

they were pleasing to the eye. It didn't

even matter if they were happy or healthy.

It wasn't the beholders that sparked my

curiosity rather what they would give me

for appearing sexy too. I had become

vain, like my father, with low self-worth,

Journey to Holistic Wellness & Weight Loss and honestly placed a very small value on other people. Everyone looked like a dollar bill, or a way to come up from my current situation.

Now in my early 20s, over 200lbs at 5'2, and clearly not healthy inside or out, a more environmental challenge became very aware. I was now able to shop for my own attire, and soon would face the struggles of "the big girl" market;

Journey to Holistic Wellness & Weight Loss most people call this industry the plus sized market. Almost every store selling women's clothing sold attire that inspired her to feel and look sexy and 'thin'. Popular clothing stores sold the most

beautiful feminine outfits in small and petite sizes, as opposed to plus sizes. Clothing for larger women, despite the age, resembled 'old lady' clothing, and embodied fewer desirable colors. I came across unappealing shades of black, grey,

brown, and darker tones when searching

the racks, not vibrant and feminine colors

like pastels or brights like in the smaller

size sections. Now of course, this is all

my own opinion but the young women I

knew, who were plus sized like me, all had

similar complaints and hated the thought

of using the dressing rooms to try on

clothes. It seemed as whoever was at the

66

head of the fashion market had decided it

was best to hide a curvy, plus sized,

woman in dark shaded colors. If you have

been considered a plus sized diva then you

may relate to what I'm saying. The

clothing options for larger women were

designed with less than tasteful patterns as

well. Different prints, and the materials

used were not as sensual, soft, pretty, or

appealing as the junior, petite, or misses

sizes were. I almost felt like the animal

prints I loved made me look more like

huge prey in a jungle, than a fiery

confident diva on the hunt for success. On

top of all these challenges the plus sized

clothes were not cut well, they didn't

accentuate my curves, and often made me

look bigger, and rounder. I was really

embarrassed by how I was forming, and

grew to hate shopping for clothing,

Journey to Holistic Wellness & Weight Loss especially intimates, swimwear, or evening wear. I had fallen for the stereotype that no man or woman, whatever your preference, would want to see all my giggly flesh in a sexy lingerie outfit, swimming at the beach, or dancing at a social event, shaking it on the dance floor. Hard on myself and lacking in self-care and self-love left me hopeless and

Journey to Holistic Wellness & Weight Loss anxiety began to knock on my door with full force! I simply had enough of living, and silently considered the opposite. With having a poor family system, a lack of support, being a dark-skinned black woman in a country run by (lighter) patriarchal systems, no higher education of learning, unhealthy and addictive eating habits, declining self-esteem issues, my virginity gone, and yeah, the guy too at this point, disassociation with my church

Journey to Holistic Wellness & Weight Loss values, and a long surmounting list of cons, I was dead inside. You can hear the despair in my voice. I was caught in a web of self-loathing and a hate for the life I had been dealt with.

Amazingly something hidden deep in me still wanted to fight, wanted to prove them all wrong, wanted a victory story not just for me but for my children someday, and all the other women silently

Journey to Holistic Wellness & Weight Loss
fighting the same battles. I knew deep down inside there was a bigger meaning for my struggles and I had to know why. I started combing through the societal system of marketing, a lack of public knowledge, and the obvious non-exposure to helpful resources. I was guided to unlock a mystery. I had matured over the years working in the world, among women and men, with very different views than the one's I had been raised with. It was

Journey to Holistic Wellness & Weight Loss there that I began seeing things from a higher perspective. My focus was re-directed after hearing and listening to other women I encountered in groups online and in books, their hearing stories of survival, how they were overcoming obstacles like abuse and addictions, and paving their own way. I realized I wasn't alone in this fight for holistic wellness and cultural freedom. There were so many other men and women, young and old,

Journey to Holistic Wellness & Weight Loss
who had experienced similar upbringing and faced similar self-esteem issues as I did. Yet, they were not afraid, or ashamed of speaking out about it publicly whether by writing self-help books, or joining motivational speaking events, in person or online.

I embarked on a whole community of activists because I had a thirst for a better understanding of who I was and

Journey to Holistic Wellness & Weight Loss
why I existed. Deep inside I loved myself enough to hold on to an energy I couldn't even see but I felt. Life had a meaning for me and I was determined to find it and utilize the hell out of it! *Side note* and real talk... As I was writing this book, I turned on my television to check the weather, and the news was broadcasting a study of how weight loss is connected to sleeping patterns, including a lack of sleep. Since obesity leads to depression,

Journey to Holistic Wellness & Weight Loss
anxiety, and an imbalance in the body of course would negatively affect how one sleeps or doesn't! Yet they failed to mention the underlying causes and instead focused on the outcome. It's currently 2023 and we are still so consumed by body image; the media is still using its platforms to 'body-shame' and promote fear using weight as a major tool. Of course, they added information that directed the viewer to solutions like diet

Journey to Holistic Wellness & Weight Loss programs and even a new and upcoming weight loss drug. This country still uses fear tactics to gain profit without truly addressing a growing issue, poor diet, and a lack of available options to good whole foods that are nutrient-based and fulfilling. I am still astonished at the boldness of it all and how subliminally they believe people are clueless about the real causes of disease and the causal factors. Turning on the television to find out what's going on

Journey to Holistic Wellness & Weight Loss
in the world, keep up with current news,

and be a participating member of society

led me right to being triggered, first thing

in the morning. Yes, although I have

come a long way to getting back to loving

myself and not being misled by societal

concepts of what I should look like, or any

woman, I still get triggered by the obvious

attempts for the media to financially

benefit off the challenges that people

battle every day, without providing

Journey to Holistic Wellness & Weight Loss realistic, attainable, and long-term solutions that don't require loads of money, cosmetic surgery, or starvation. Personally, I know so many women who have suffered permanent scars, mental and emotional anguish, and huge financial loss due to trying to follow a systematic flow of marketed weight loss solutions, not formulated to each woman's individual needs, limiting their long-term success.

Journey to Holistic Wellness & Weight Loss
Back to what led to my solution.

After years of exposure to birth control, weight loss diets/drinks, and other prescribed and non-prescribed medicines to treat of load of health issues and combat their own side effects causing huge hormonal influxes that led to even more weight gain, and depression I finally dropped the ball on all of it! I found that my hair was thinning over time, my skin suffered from rashes and dry patches, and

Journey to Holistic Wellness & Weight Loss
I wasn't reaching my desired weight goal

anyway. I was always moody and

remained hungry, and I often experienced

digestion issues; not to mention what

drugs, and diet schemes did for to my

libido. I just wanted to look and feel

'normal', live in a healthy body, and I was

desperate to end the pain. So, I said to

myself (F) it all. I really craved

acceptance, compassion, and love but I

was over waiting for life to deliver it to

Journey to Holistic Wellness & Weight Loss
my door. Why couldn't anyone notice me

and the suffering going on within me.

Was I so unloved or broken for anyone to

love? By the age of 23 I weighed over

225 lbs. You can imagine the weight had

caused a hopelessness that only led to

more weight gain and by 25 I was 285lbs

and now suffering from health issues

related to being obese like asthma, high

blood pressure, arthritis, and pre-diabetes.

My parents didn't even address it or think

Journey to Holistic Wellness & Weight Loss
of getting me the overall health care I
obviously needed at this point. I don't
even think they recognized that I had
spiraled out of control. I found it was not
a thing black people did, therapy that is.
Seeing a psychiatrist or psychologist was
taboo in many urban communities, and it
still is today. Obesity was considered a
condition of greed and not a real disease
(addiction) requiring medical attention. I
was belittled and blamed for my inability

to maintain a healthy weight by choosing good options in moderate portions. In other words, I was seen as greedy and undisciplined. As a food addict this made recovery nearly impossible, you wouldn't place drug addicts seeking recovery in an environment full of drug dealers and easy access to narcotics, then shame them for not being able to beat temptation, unless your motive is to keep them a slave to needing you for survival. My daily food

Journey to Holistic Wellness & Weight Loss options at home, and outside, included foods cooked in heavy oils, high calorie processed ingredients, chemicals like additives that aid in skin disorders, and energy stealing meals. No one cared to consider my diet as the cause of my weight issues. I hadn't learned what healthy eating looked or tasted like at home or in public, not at school or church, and coming from a deep Southern background you know we ate like fat cats.

Journey to Holistic Wellness & Weight Loss
We often had foods like fried chicken, beef soaked in gravy, white rice, loaded pasta dishes, all our greens were cooked with pork fat, the corn sweetened with sugar, yams and white potatoes at every celebration, mac-n-cheese was a staple, home baked breads, and scrumptious desserts, etc., you get it. Mouthwatering to hear but debilitating consequences would follow from eating this way for years. My mom was a great baker so there were

Journey to Holistic Wellness & Weight Loss always cakes, cookies, and pies readily available; a kitchen witch of sorts for those who know the southern way. I was doomed from the start to be overweight, unhealthy, and constantly searching for answers to lose weight. The responsibility eventually became all mine because the success of reaching a ripe old age was slowly diminishing every day. No one was lifting the fork to my mouth, no one was going to take my body outside for a

Journey to Holistic Wellness & Weight Loss
walk, no one was going to attend support

groups, or invest in better eating habits for

me. All I had was myself to blame, at this

point going forward. It was time to take

responsibility and stop crying over spilled

milk.

Even though I was medically

considered obese, by (European) standards

I obtained my first permanent, full-time

job working in the retail industry. I was

Journey to Holistic Wellness & Weight Loss placed where I didn't have to be in the front office. I felt this placement was so I could blend in more with all the other 'heavy set people'. It appeared more and more that the plus sized community was strategically hidden as opposed to having the opportunity to stand out. I worked in a large retail store in the miss's department folding clothes all day. Working long hours, and now also attending college (yes, I eventually entered college life),

Journey to Holistic Wellness & Weight Loss guess what I ate on the go, fast foods, and a lot of coffee. It was the only thing made available on my college campus. Every morning, I stopped at Dunkin donuts or Starbucks for an extra-large flavored coffee and a breakfast sandwich, or bakery item. Lunch was more of the same. A large amount of my income went to eating outside; I had to eat for energy. I decided to apply for a credit card to save my cash supply for immediate needs like food,

Journey to Holistic Wellness & Weight Loss
toiletries, hobbies etc. Only manifesting

more problems and more bills. I didn't

even have it in me anymore to ask for help

or know where I could get it, it was just

me, myself, and I at this point. I still lived

at home so rent and utilities were not an

issue, thankfully! Days turned into weeks,

weeks into months, and months into years

and I was simply going with the flow. But

was I truly addressing anything? I had

decided to accept the life I had been giving

Journey to Holistic Wellness & Weight Loss
but I think I had just given up altogether.

I had stopped going out much and had

disconnected with most of my friends.

Life was living and people often took

different directions, losing connection.   I

went from work to home and back again

for the next couple of years.

Hallelujah! There is a God.....

One bright sunny season, life

through me a lucky coin and I met a man

Journey to Holistic Wellness & Weight Loss y'all! I felt comfortable in my own skin because I knew he had met me at my heaviest weight and still wanted to love and hold me. We spent a lot of time together talking about our goals and the future, it felt so good to have someone see me. After college, we got engaged and soon after we got married. "I is married now!" (quote from the Color Purple) I remember thinking how wrong my father was. Someone did love me just the way I

Journey to Holistic Wellness & Weight Loss was. enough to marry. *I didn't feel the need to drag out the entire history of how we met and became lovers and eventually married, this book isn't a romance novel.*

It was finally time to break away from home. It was the beginning of a life I could guide on my own terms. I soon wanted to start my own family. I needed lots of love in my life. Unfortunately, the side effects from years of taking birth control pills led to me miscarrying twice.

Journey to Holistic Wellness & Weight Loss
Did you just sigh? I know, I know, more pain, misfortune, and loss. My hormones were all over the place, my overall health was not optimal for childbirth. I hadn't addressed my weight and other health issues. Happy that I had found love and wanting to secure it I was eager to give him a child. Newly married, there was still the insecurity that he would one day wake and see me for real. I couldn't run from my reality, or mask it with the love

Journey to Holistic Wellness & Weight Loss from outside of me. I was always waiting for the day that my husband would notice all my flaws, and leave. We were still young and although we spoke of it often, we really didn't have a solid plan, and neither of us came from homes that consisted of parents that had learned to live outside of society's conformities. We were winging it and hoping for the best. So, as you probably guessed, the marriage didn't last long, he did cheat with a

Journey to Holistic Wellness & Weight Loss
woman of much lesser weight than I. The
other woman became pregnant with his
first born instead of me, I was shattered
inside. Had I manifested everything that
was happening through my insecurities
and co-dependent energy? I know you
thought it was smooth sailing there for a
while. lol. God was punishing me for
some past life sin, I just knew this was for
sure. What was I going to do? I wasn't
running back home with a divorce

Journey to Holistic Wellness & Weight Loss
pending. I wouldn't give my family the

benefit of being right. Who could I run to

for help. It seemed the world had chosen

to see me as a stain on life.   Dating was

out of the question, neither was hanging

out with friends I had met while married.

I shamefully didn't want to be in the

public eye, and I didn't even want to eat;

starving   myself   also   proved

counterproductive, I soon realized. Now

28 years old, already married, and

Journey to Holistic Wellness & Weight Loss
divorced wat was next for me.   Despite

my obvious weight issue, I would have

been considered a good catch.   I had a

college degree, secured my own studio

apartment, had no children yet, and was

self-sufficient, except for the mounting

credit debt, can't win them all. Seemingly

a good catch, right but who had the desire

to catch such a big fish!

Journey to Holistic Wellness & Weight Loss
Are you ready to take a turn for the better with me, finally! On a wintery, wrapped in a blanket drinking coffee, my addiction, I scrolled through the internet searching for weight lost miracles. I had tried everything from Weight Watchers, Jenny Craig, diet pills and powders to those expensive gym memberships that I never used, consistently. Fasting and detoxing felt more like torturing and starving myself, only to binge right after. I

Journey to Holistic Wellness & Weight Loss

bought expensive in-home exercise equipment that ended up collecting dust or served as a place to dry laundry on. Desperate for support and community I joined online groups promoting weight loss unity, only to see members drop off for being bullied by other members; the world can be a cruel place. *Okay, now stay with me through this next part and keep an open mind please!* I came across a man named Dr. Sebi, he has since passed

Journey to Holistic Wellness & Weight Loss

away. He spoke about food in a way I had never heard before.   What intrigued me the most about his approach was that food portions were not restricted, at all, and the food was readily available in my local supermarket for reasonable prices.   I realized, I truly did not know or understand food, and how to shop for it. The lifestyle he promoted, and yes, I said lifestyle (NOT DIET) seemed the most realistic form of weight loss and healthy

Journey to Holistic Wellness & Weight Loss

living that I had heard, ever. Skeptical still, I began to read all the success stories posted by thousands of people, even celebrities. I found myself growing more and more curious about the things he said, unlike many other diet plans that turned me off immediately. Now hopeful, I believed that this lifestyle change might work. There was nothing to lose by trying, except the weight. *Now, those of you that know Dr. Sebi might already want*

Journey to Holistic Wellness & Weight Loss

to stop reading but believe me you don't want to do that just yet! I utilized most of his approach but found I could tweak it here and there, to fit my life and weight loss goals better. I found that with any dietary goal there is always room to make it work for you with simple changes that won't impede you from losing the weight you seek.

Journey to Holistic Wellness & Weight Loss

****At this point, I will digress for just a moment, and highly recommend that you get a full physical to check your hormonal levels, and overall health to ensure success in achieving any weight loss goal. It is very important to maintain your overall health regardless of trying to lose weight. Nothing written in this text supersedes seeking medical attention when needed, and it all comes from my own opinion and experience. ****

Journey to Holistic Wellness & Weight Loss

Make sure you are giving attention to your body, in a holistic way, and that you are not just focused on quick fixed ideas that won't last long term. I now understand that nutrition and diet is a lifestyle and not a project. I now realized that because my eating habits were acquired and learned by societal, generational, and cultural systems that were guiding my poor choices, and the belief in how I should feed myself I had to

Journey to Holistic Wellness & Weight Loss

limit my exposure to temptation. I had a lot of years of conditioning to release, and work through. My attachment to food was more than just a taste for flavor, it was a chemically reactive need to give my body what it had been used to receiving consistently for a lifetime, a co-dependency. I had learned to see eating as a reward system, and not as a means of survival. I was taught that you ate what you were given, without any mindful

Journey to Holistic Wellness & Weight Loss

thought, and showed gratitude for the fact that it was prepared, cooked, and supplied by God and my elders. I didn't dare question how it was prepared, if the preparation was done with the utmost health benefit in mind, or if the proportions I received were intended to sustain a healthy body weight. My parents cooked as their parents cooked but took it up a notch to show that their financial status had been upgraded from a poverty

Journey to Holistic Wellness & Weight Loss

mindset. This mindset slowly but surely became a recipe for obesity and disease and illnesses that would be passed down for generations to come. The belief is disease and illness passed on through our children are hereditary and acquired through generational DNA. My belief is that what is hereditary, by way of your culture's eating habits, causes diseases to continually manifest in your generations; we are what we eat. If heart disease,

Journey to Holistic Wellness & Weight Loss

diabetes, cancer, hypertension etc. runs in your family, take a hard look at how the lineages are being fed! That's just to name a few diseases and or illnesses that have a strong connection to what we put into our bodies.

Fast forwarding, I was now a mother of three, on my third husband, working a full-time job, juggling to provide and survive, multi-tasking. I

Journey to Holistic Wellness & Weight Loss

incorporated his instructions, and most of Dr. Sebi's wisdom. I started on a journey to changing my eating habits and adopted a pescatarian lifestyle, at first. Meat was never really something that agreed with my gut so I started slowly deleting certain meats from my meals and replaced them with more nutritional, and still delicious choices like fish. I changed the condiments I used in cooking for seasoning and flavoring dishes, and I

Journey to Holistic Wellness & Weight Loss

learned what foods not to eat together to decrease insulin spikes, diabetes wreaked havoc in my family. I learned about how to replace fatty oils with broths when cooking and would bake, sauté, and broil when possible, eliminating frying, and fatty bases. Ditching my deep fryer for an air fryer to cut out the fat was life changing. I created my own healthy treats and enjoyed inventing new dishes with my children. Cooking became fun and

Journey to Holistic Wellness & Weight Loss

adventurous and I was surprised to see how creative I could be. I took full control of what I put in my mouth and how I would feed my family, and the many generations to come from the lives I started; to many this is equal to the concept of breaking generational curses. I knew I had the task of healing myself and thus helping to heal those coming after me, and I took that seriously. How could I be okay with irresponsibly shoveling food

Journey to Holistic Wellness & Weight Loss

into the mouths of my children and claiming I loved them, even though what I was feeding them could bring them years of battling disease and challenging health issues? Eating well was about something bigger than myself, a concept I had wished my parents mentally embraced. Don't get me wrong? I never blamed my parents for my issues with weight, directly. I understood that coming from a scarcity mindset in the 1940s through the 1970s

Journey to Holistic Wellness & Weight Loss

left them hoarding and indulging in the pleasure of becoming financially independent and living a middle-class lifestyle at all costs. My parents were both descendants of slavery and watched their parents struggle to provide for their families. They did the best they could with the belief that they were giving more to their children, than they had. I do not remember a time when portion control was

Journey to Holistic Wellness & Weight Loss routinely used in my home, growing up.

A

child who blew up years later after consuming, indulging, and grossly accumulating food was now my responsibility to cure. Although I saw it coming, I could have done little to stop it and decided to forgive myself, and my parents. Any who, enough of the nostalgia, let's sink into resolution-based

Journey to Holistic Wellness & Weight Loss information, shall we? As I said, Dr. Sebi had finally suggested a plan that was doable and there was no reason I couldn't

achieve my goal. There was an even greater advantage to incorporating his ideology, the minimal amount of physical exercise it would take for me to see real results! *Yes, of course, adding exercise is optimal for any weight loss journey and will most likely shorten the time it will take*

Journey to Holistic Wellness & Weight Loss
to lose weight, and make you feel stronger

along the way. Unfortunately, my weight

early in my process made it more difficult

to work out every day. I was a very busy

single mother and time was always an

issue; thus, eating on the run. Let's be real

though. Being obese, as the doctors called

it, makes exercise not only challenging

and difficult but it is often a huge deterrent

for many fighting the battle to lose weight.

Journey to Holistic Wellness & Weight Loss
Therefore, having an achievable plan with

minimal exertion, especially from the

start, was very appealing.

My overall concept was based in

eating a variety of whole plant-based

foods that would not only balance my

hormones, which at this point were all

over the place, and allow me to feel

satisfied. It needed to re-teach my body to

Journey to Holistic Wellness & Weight Loss maintain a healthy weight and feel greater

as time went on. Yep, it was possible and

doable without feeling starved or punished

or continuously counting calories

throughout the day. Who has time for

that? I was conditioned to love to eat, it's

true, and I didn't want to feel guilty about

it. I worked and earned my own way and

felt I deserved to eat happily. So, the first

thing I did was slow down when having a

Journey to Holistic Wellness & Weight Loss
meal, remembering to take my time and give my body time to digest and absorb my meal fully. I made a list of my favorite things to eat, itemized them categorically, and sat with my list, making changes when necessary to feel satisfied. This helped me

see which food groups I ate the most and why or how they affected my overall health. It was no surprise that it was

Journey to Holistic Wellness & Weight Loss
carbohydrates that took the win. For years

I was prone to buying and eating bread,

rice, pasta, cookies, pastries, and lots of

baked sweets!   I realized that it was

important, to achieve my goal, I had to be

honest about the work that needed to be

done. I had to admit all my flaws, habits,

and negative self-talk and take

accountability for what I was shoveling

into my mouth without being forced. I

Journey to Holistic Wellness & Weight Loss owned it, every embarrassing, harsh, and painful revelation. Meditating and sitting with my higher self-brought a lot of tears, shame, compassion, judgement, love, and soon all the negative talking ceased. My body had craved carbohydrates and sugary foods not only because, obviously, they tasted delicious lol, but because I had been consuming them for so long, consistently.

Journey to Holistic Wellness & Weight Loss
I had programmed my brain to need the constant fix, sugar was my drug of choice. I wasn't greedy, I wasn't careless, I was addicted! I knew I had to focus on treating the addiction to program my mind to choose healthier options that fulfilled my desire for taste, and reward. Yes, I said reward. Most people who indulge in unhealthy food choices can chop it up to an excuse to reward oneself after a long work week, surviving a stressful situation,

Journey to Holistic Wellness & Weight Loss
socializing with friends, overcoming a life obstacle and so on, you get it. What is not considered is, is it really a reward if it causes harmful, unhealthy illness and disease, or contributes to weight gain and thus low self-esteem and depression? Terms like reward, treat, earned, deserved, etc. are just triggered responses for hidden shame, guilt, remorse, or the ego etc. It felt better to come up with some fictional reason that was giving me permission to

Journey to Holistic Wellness & Weight Loss

eat whatever I wanted, regardless of consequence, then to truly discern why I couldn't say no. It didn't help that the same people who had no problem pointing out my weight, as if I didn't own a mirror, also had no problem offering me horrible food choices when I visited their homes. Yeah, I know they didn't spoon feed it to me and I could have said no thank you! But do we blame an addict for relapsing after we offer them the drugs wrapped up

Journey to Holistic Wellness & Weight Loss
with a bow? Do we blame an alcoholic

for taking a drink when it is offered to

them in a well-chilled glass by a person

who they believe loves them? Sugar has

the same effects as alcohol on the brain.

Carbohydrates are just another form of

sugar, when broken down in the body. It

is a matter of educating yourself and not

simply accepting the ideas of ideas. Fast

foods contain massive amounts of carbs

i.e. French fries, breads/wraps/buns as

Journey to Holistic Wellness & Weight Loss associated with pizza, burgers, quesadillas.

Sugary sauces like BBQ, teriyaki, ketchup, and syrup on pancakes, waffles were made available in every restaurant. All the added ingredients in breakfast cereals, hot or cold, bagels, donuts, muffins, and croissants added pounds of weight and caused skin irritants. Corn and vegetable (soy) oils were heavily used in all households when cooking leading to heart disease, a number one killer in the US.

Journey to Holistic Wellness & Weight Loss
Many coffee shops offering highly sweetened and flavored beverages had been placed in every neighborhood not far from atm machines and a place to sit and enjoy. Most of these food choices we consume as daily options for on-the-go quick meals and in multiple quantities. It might be okay to eat these treats in moderation but who is counting anyway when life is a never-ending race against time, but time for what? We are busy just

Journey to Holistic Wellness & Weight Loss trying to make it through the day to return home, only to consume some more and sit on our comfy couch or lay in our bed relieved that the day is done.

Now, fast-forwarding into 2023, with door-to-door delivery services like Door Dash, Uber Eats, Grubhub etc. who must cook? Pizza Hut, Papa Johns, and Dominoes will quickly feed the whole family after a hard day's work for pennies

Journey to Holistic Wellness & Weight Loss

on the dollar compared to grocery shopping. We can grab a bucket of chicken at Popeyes, or KFC including side options or speed through the drive through at McDonalds or Burger King. There's Wing Stop, Shake Shack, Chinese takeout, and we even get bamboozled ordering salads filled with toppings like croutons, bacon, fried chicken, BBQ meats, sour cream, cheese blends and heavy oil-based or sugary dressings. Once again, these

Journey to Holistic Wellness & Weight Loss options are acceptable in moderation but are we really checking? Are the choices they provide cooked in a healthy way or are they geared for a much bigger plan? I know you may be thinking "wow that's a lot to consider, you just want to eat" but don't you also want to LIVE a well and healthy long life? One that's free of illness and disease that may have plagued your family for generations. Even more important, don't you want to protect the

Journey to Holistic Wellness & Weight Loss generations that come from and are attached to you? I've seen mothers, fathers, grandparents and so on bury their children, grandchildren, and those so much younger than they, who pass away from childhood diseases related to poor diets causing obesity, diabetes, heart disease, cancer etc. Yes, cancer too can be connected to dietary intake like consuming carcinogens in meats and cooking procedures that include artery blocking

Journey to Holistic Wellness & Weight Loss
oils etc. No parent should bury their child,

especially if it was preventable by making

some simple life changes.

On another note, to relieve you of

some of the personal consequences of

making healthy food choices, let's address

the economic cost of eating healthy vs not.

I understand the difficulties faced when

shopping at the markets for affordable

healthy foods to feed a growing family. I

Journey to Holistic Wellness & Weight Loss
have shopped for years and years for not only myself, but also my children and at one time my spouse. This left me with the burden of having a lot of responsibility for the foods they ate and how their health was eventually affected. I shopped, prepared, cooked, and served my whole family daily with foods they would eat early in the mornings on the weekend, and at night before bed.   How they nutritionally started and ended each day

Journey to Holistic Wellness & Weight Loss was navigated by me. I used my family's overall appearance to navigate how I examined my ability to know food. I could imagine the next generation of diseases looming as I watched society feed itself and it kept me on target with my goals. I had to interrupt the external challenges to good health and replace them with positive models. I had to get inspired to create a positive, loving, and nutritionally good environment for everyone I had an

Journey to Holistic Wellness & Weight Loss
obligation to care for, by being intentional.

My family was my inspiration to holistic

wellness but if you don't have children or

a mate to prepare meals for, aren't you

enough? When that beautiful family

becomes a part of your life you could

already have done the work to be an

inspiration of good health practices.

Okay, so where did all these

emotions, reflections, and self-awareness

Journey to Holistic Wellness & Weight Loss take me? I broke down my eating habits, my choices when cooking, categorized my daily intake based on my moods, meditated, and kept a journal daily of how I was doing emotionally and physically, got a yearly health check to look for deficiencies or monitor changes in my body, SLOWED DOWN especially when eating, and focused on nutritional intake vs quantity.   Carbohydrates, proteins, dairy, sugars, fruits and vegetables,

Journey to Holistic Wellness & Weight Loss beverages, snacks, and condiments were my top categories. I came up with carbs, sugars, and dairy as being my go-to options daily; this is where my det needed to most changes. Then on fruits and veggies which came out on the bottom; proteins were somewhat in the middle. I was never a person who had to have meat with every meal but I did choose a sweet treat, bread, rice, or potato option for breakfast, lunch, and dinner. Then I

Journey to Holistic Wellness & Weight Loss
decided which led to good or bad health,

that was easy! I then decided which items

I could replace with a healthier option but

not replace the taste or satisfaction factor,

this proved a bit more challenging. I used

Dr. Sebi's food group list when it came to

healthier fruit and vegetables options and

how to prepare them to get the most

nutrients from them. I watched countless

videos and disciplined myself to get more

educated in holistic wellness. I replaced

Journey to Holistic Wellness & Weight Loss wasted hours watching reality tv or some other useless forms of passing my extra time with gaining knowledge of my body, how food worked for or against it, and how to prepare dishes in healthier ways to truly care for it. As a woman especially it was important to check my blood and hormone levels knowing these have a huge factor in how we are formed over the years, having children, menstrual cycles, and thus menopause. Men and women

Journey to Holistic Wellness & Weight Loss carry weight in very different ways and it should be respected and added to a holistic wellness routine. Starting from a clean slate, a healthy outlook, and a realistic goal made all the difference. The mind is a powerful thing and we can self-sabotage ourselves simply by subscribing to pre-existing negative self-talk, shaming, guilt, denial, overthinking, and a fear of failure before we even get started. I paid close attention to how I spoke to my inner self

Journey to Holistic Wellness & Weight Loss
and incorporated a daily regimen of self-affirmations and journaling my goals, challenges, and achievements in my process to losing weight, becoming healthier, and changing my life forever. I bought affirmation cards and kept them in my pocketbook to pull and read during my day at work. I kept sticky notes to jot down any mood changes, or reminders of how a certain food made my energy rise or fall throughout the day. I read more

Journey to Holistic Wellness & Weight Loss healing self-help books and added a little 'erotica' every now and then. This helped boost my libido, chakras, aura, and feminine energy, and thus stabilize my hormones too. I also purchased coloring books, puzzle books, and took up crochet as a form of healthy distraction when craving old habits, this helped alleviate moments of open windows for snacking and being bored. I found doing something with my physical hands other than playing

Journey to Holistic Wellness & Weight Loss games on my phone disciplined my brain muscle, and alleviated the need for hand-to-mouth movements, a double benefit. You'd be surprised how little you control your movements daily!

I took the unhealthy options like sugary snacks, beverages, and carbohydrates (that broke down to sugar in the body) and replaced them with naturally sweet fruits and created my own snacks

Journey to Holistic Wellness & Weight Loss
like cookies and candies using dried fruits

adding seeds and nuts. I ate them fresh or

by baking them. I created options like

sliced candied rolls from oatmeal quinoa,

buckwheat, chia seed, flax seed, added

nuts, fruits etc. I made my own healthy

chips from plantains, bananas, and yuca

using sea salt or Himalayan salts and

healthier oils for lightly frying like

grapeseed or sesame seed; but air frying is

the best option any day to crisp anything!

Journey to Holistic Wellness & Weight Loss

I opted for loaded salads with fresh organic whole food ingredients, not including processed ingredients like croutons. I could add my proteins to my salad like salmon, tuna, avocado, pasture raised eggs, and I always included lots of fresh veggies like romaine, spinach, arugula, kale, sprouts, cucumber, tomato, peppers, mushrooms, green onions, sprouts, arugula, mint, parsley, basil, cilantro, edamame, beans like chickpeas or

Journey to Holistic Wellness & Weight Loss
black beans, beets, celery, red cabbage etc.

I mixed and matched and always had a brand-new salad creation waiting. I made my salads pleasing to the eye (we eat what we see, as pleasing, colorful, and this also was beneficial in getting the whole family to enjoy them, it kept them curious about what the next dish would look like and taste like. If you have young children to feed you know the benefits of what a colorful, fragrant, multi-textured meal

Journey to Holistic Wellness & Weight Loss could have on their choices, to eat. I knew my food had to have desirable textures like crunchy, or chewy, or firm mixed in my salads to trick my mind into thinking I was eating meat or enjoying a snack when I was simply eating a salad full of veggies. I included things like seeds, nuts, whole fruit and dried fruits, air fried veggies, plant-based proteins etc. My kids often couldn't tell if they were having a dessert or a healthy meal. I learned to make my own treats in a healthier way like cookies,

candies, pastries, breads, etc. by using

organic whole ingredients and air frying or

baking or even using a dehydrator to make

dried fruits without the added sugars and

oils. I purchased a nut milk machine and

stopped giving my family chemically

processed, hormonally enhanced, and

inflammation building cow milk. That

was my main reason for choosing to breast

feed my babies from the start of their

Journey to Holistic Wellness & Weight Loss young lives. Yet as they were off, they became slaves to dairy products at school and at home.

Soon the whole family was excited about what the next treat, or creative dish would be and the children volunteered to help in the kitchen, with all the new and fun gadgets. I was teaching the next generation how to prepare healthy, delicious, fun meals without asking,

Journey to Holistic Wellness & Weight Loss
begging, or fooling them into eating well.

We began making grocery shopping day
an event where everyone got to choose a
dish they wanted to try and find the
ingredients; they were learning to navigate
the market with an eye for nutrition as
opposed to an eye to satisfy an insatiable
addiction, or bad habit, choosing sugary,
processed, and a high fat foods and treats.
Not only were we focused on healthier
living, but we were also looking out for

Journey to Holistic Wellness & Weight Loss
each other, and building loving connections. I could see the weight falling off and I felt proud of myself and then my self-esteem improved greatly. I began to put more intention in getting outside, going for nature walks, sitting in a quiet meditation, reading good books, taking better care of my overall appearance like my hair and skin; everything was improving and it almost seemed effortless.

Journey to Holistic Wellness & Weight Loss
Drinking water was always a challenging task for me. I didn't like the taste of most bottled waters, and was careful not to drink tap water, ever! After sampling many brands, I found bottled water that finally satisfied my taste buds. Consuming more water in juices led me to using my juicer more; this really boosted my weight loss, increased hydration for skin health, and increased my energy. I made sure to try and find organic fruits

Journey to Holistic Wellness & Weight Loss
and veggies to juice and cut down on chemicals added to my food sources. Nearly all my meals were freshly made, always satisfying, and I could change the ingredients every day. I eventually couldn't live without juicing; right from my home conveniently and way cheaper than grabbing a juice from the health store. I washed and prepped my veggies and fruits and placed them in freezer baggies to grab, juice, and go. The children also

Journey to Holistic Wellness & Weight Loss began to juice making theirs taste like milkshakes and smoothies, without the bad stuff. We went from juicing to a high-speed blender to making dressings, pancake and waffles mixes, and even hot soups right in the processor. I bought everyone their own-colored storage bottles to take delicious, healthy beverages to school, work, or just outside enjoying a nature day and play with friends. Every bottle was packed with nature's vitamins,

Journey to Holistic Wellness & Weight Loss
minerals, and healthy fat burning ingredients, naturally! My children's friends even started asking about their drinks and wanted to try them, they were so colorful and looked like sweet treats to the kids. Some even contained healthy gut ingredients like non-dairy yogurt with probiotics. I also included power foods like sea moss, chia seed, hemp seed, flax seed, soursop, pomegranate, etc. to boost the minerals and increase the benefits of

Journey to Holistic Wellness & Weight Loss
the juice. Also, there are seeds that promote weight loss and chia is one of them. The juice was not only providing a huge source of nutrition it was providing lots of water, adding to the weight loss by burning fat while restoring vitamins, and minerals. I began to see fat turn into muscle which and I learned to food prep for convenience and to save time. We were all enjoying our new lifestyle and it was showing in our mental, emotional, -

Journey to Holistic Wellness & Weight Loss
and physical behaviors.   The road to

weight loss went from being a nightmare

to a positive and rewarding experience for

my whole family. I learned that it doesn't

have to cost a ton of money, consist of

torturous diet schemes, counting every

calorie, expensive gym memberships,

unnecessary   surgery,   embarrassing

counseling sessions, or self-loathing fat

shaming depression. I chose to nature

walks, including opportunities to walk the

Journey to Holistic Wellness & Weight Loss
family dog, remembering to keep a and

comfortable pace doing laps around the

neighborhood or on the track in the park,

while shopping, doing household chores

like laundry and cleaning, swimming at

the local poo with the children, and

incorporating some at-home yoga in front

of the television. These low impact, free

flowing, and self-guided forms of

including exercise in my life were the only

exercise I did, and it was enjoyable, and at

Journey to Holistic Wellness & Weight Loss
my own pace, and FREE! The healthier I began to feel the more I wanted to do more things outdoors.

Soon my friends and family were all asking what I was doing. They were complimenting me on how great I started to look, and even how happier I appeared. Let me tell y'all too, the more energetic I felt the more I entertained returning to a healthy relationship, and wanted a sex life,

Journey to Holistic Wellness & Weight Loss
that was an added benefit I didn't see coming. I began to share life-saving information in my community, simply sitting with neighbors and chatting. The community around me was full of illnesses like diabetes, heart disease, cancer, thyroid disease, COPD, and skin ailments. People were really listening and watching my transformation and I was shocked and humbled by the recognition, and positive feedback. My father who was now a

Journey to Holistic Wellness & Weight Loss
diabetic and taking pills every day, getting closer to being insulin dependent, soon stopped taking the prescribed pills, after following my dietary suggestions, and saw his numbers return to healthy levels. Of course, I credited Dr. Sebi for guiding me to this new way of eating and looking at food. I stand on that statement; he changed my life forever! Remember, I utilized many of his suggestions but did tweak many of his suggestions to fit my

Journey to Holistic Wellness & Weight Loss

own needs, and those of my family as well. I was still able to achieve the benefits of his formula, in my own way. He taught me how food choices, in combination, manifested in the body after consumption. I learned which veggies were starches/carbs and how consuming certain oils and cooking with them was extremely harmful. I learned which veggies could be used for proteins and contained higher percentages of nutrition,

Journey to Holistic Wellness & Weight Loss
that could aid in breaking down body fat.

Most of all I learned it was possible to eat until I was full and satisfied all the while losing weight and burning fat without counting calories. I saw food and eating as something joyful instead of shameful and that changed my life!

All the information written in this book is manifestations of my own personal journey to self-love, self-healing, holistic

Journey to Holistic Wellness & Weight Loss wellness, and survival. Nothing written is meant to replace the need for any type of medical care, when necessary, I am not a doctor. I will say that it is a doable, healthy, self-guided, and self-empowering map to discovering your inner strength and endurance. There were times I considered giving up on life and being a part of this planet. Feeling like an outsider who wasn't worthy of love, and recognition left me defeated, and hopeless. I want you to

Journey to Holistic Wellness & Weight Loss
know if you are feeling, or ever felt tis

way THERE IS A LIGHT waiting for you

at the end of a tunnel you may not see yet!

Don't give up on having the amazingly

beautiful life that you truly deserve. We

are all made in the eyes of a merciful God

that has equipped us wit everything we

need to survive and thrive in the world.

We get distracted by the voices of others

around us through what we watch, read,

listen to, and believe. So, the key to living

Journey to Holistic Wellness & Weight Loss
your best life is to make your own voice

your own compass. Choose every day to

engross yourself in positive affirmations,

habits, people especially, and places you

visit. Give your time to what feels good

mentally, not just physically. Be the

master of your world and not a slave to

conformity. Rest more than you run

through your day, even if it's taking

breaks to meditate, breathe, and remember

you're doing your best, and in time it will

be

Journey to Holistic Wellness & Weight Loss

enough. Metaphorically speaking, if the ride you're on through life feels confusing, or void of happy stops along the way, or is steered in a direction you don't control, jump off. That's your sign that you need to seek another mode of transportation, until you arrive at a destination that brings you joy and personal freedom. Don't ever be afraid of trying a road less traveled, which is what I did trying Dr. Sebi's lifestyle and diet changes. Never be afraid

Journey to Holistic Wellness & Weight Loss

to set healthy boundaries with family and friends who bring you down wit negative energy and hateful comments, subliminally! Take your life back from a world that means to control you and keep you stuck in a daily bubble of anxiety building living. There is no one else like you in the world and you must remember how special that is. You are not your body; you are a beautiful soul meant to shine your light on this planet.

Journey to Holistic Wellness & Weight Loss

TIME TO LET IT SHINE

Be healthy….Be happy…..Be YOU…….

Suggested texts:

Dr. Sebi's Anti-inflammatory Diet

Dr. Sebi's Self-Healing Bible

Unknown author, 2024 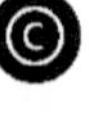

171